Take Your Medicine

Eddy Jefferson

TAKE YOUR MEDICINE EDDY JEFFERSON. THAT'S NO DRAGON IN THE SKY, THAT'S A PLANE AND YOUR BRAIN SEES THINGS THAT ARE NOT REAL LIFE.

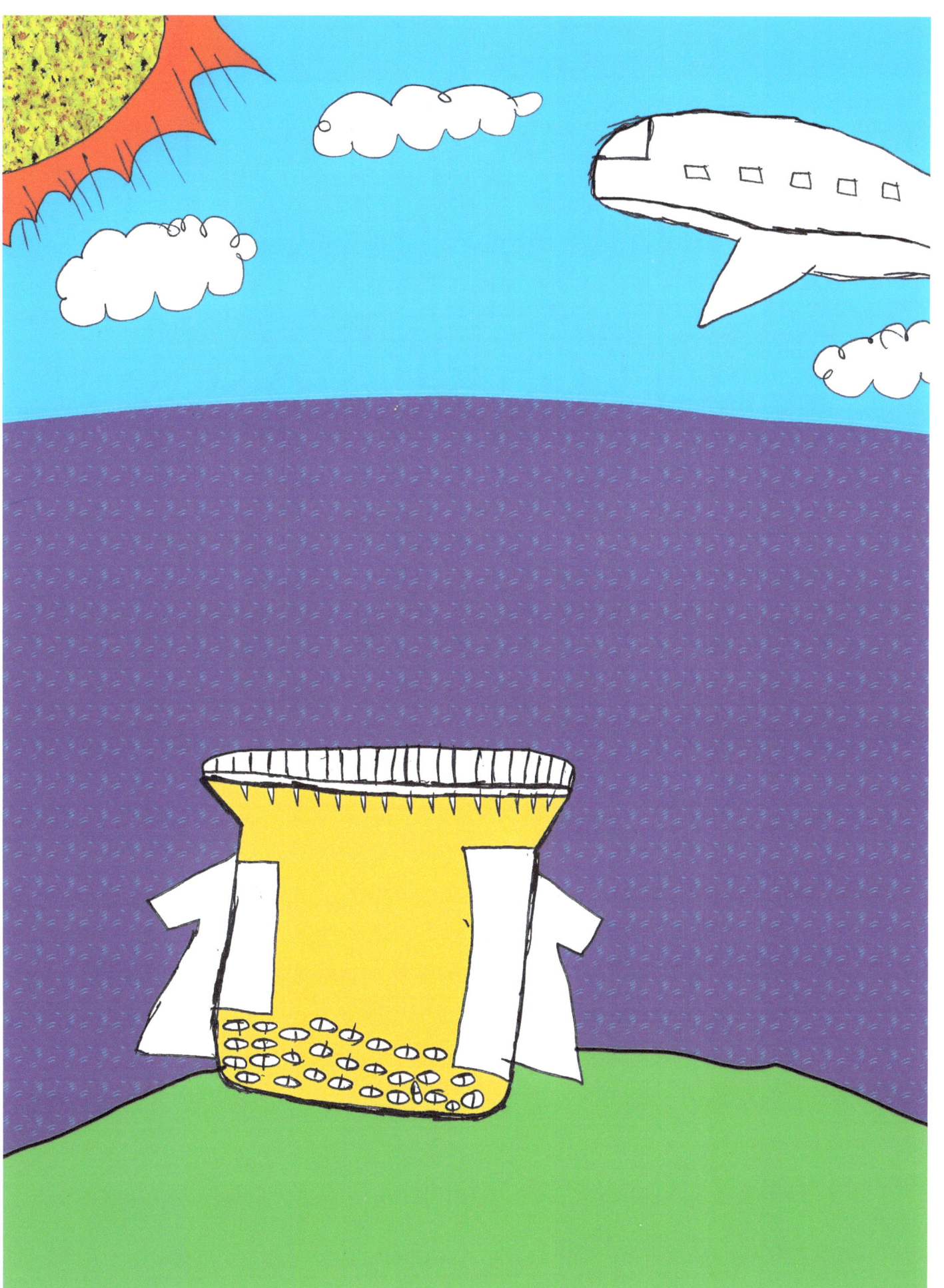

TAKE YOUR MEDICINE EDDY JEFFERSON, DON'T TAKE THIS AS A COMPLAINT. BUT YOU REALLY OUGHT TO TAKE IT, I DON'T WANT YOU IN RESTRAINTS.

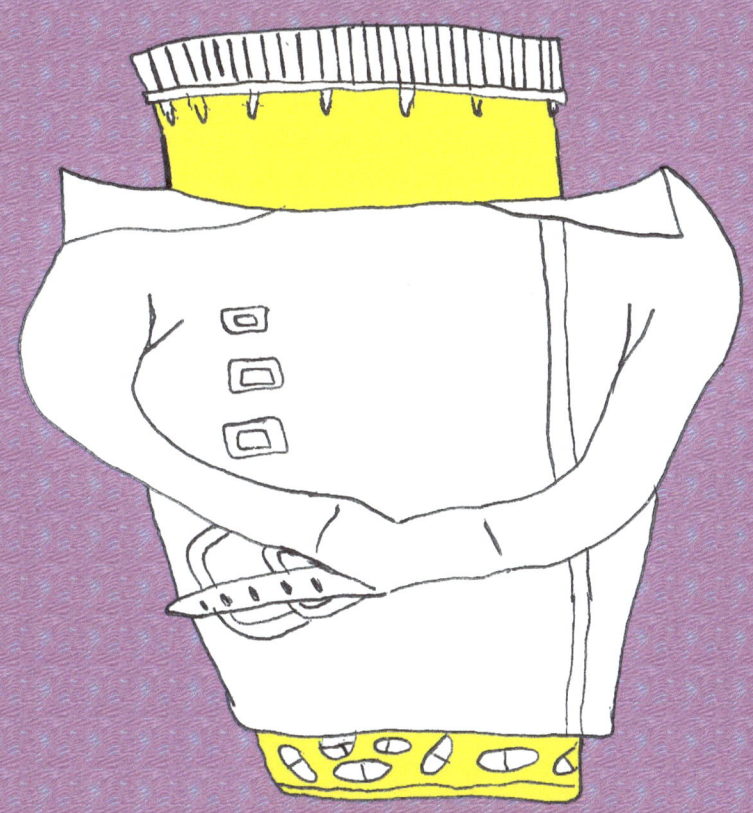

FUDGEWILLI

TAKE YOUR MEDICINE

EDDY JEFFERSON BECAUSE

THOSE VOICES ARE

UNNERVING. THEY'RE NOT

SERVING ANY PURPOSE BESIDE

BEING SO DISTURBING.

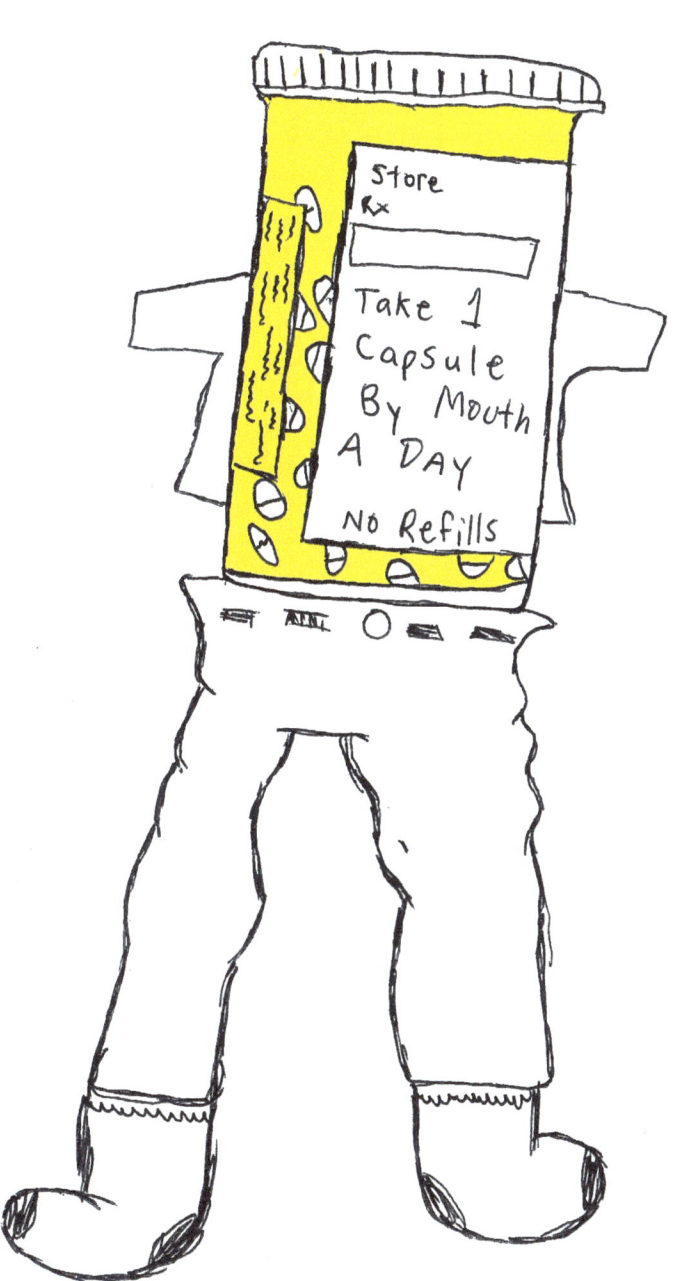

TAKE YOUR MEDICINE EDDY JEFFERSON BECAUSE YOUR SPEECH IS NOT COHERENT. AND I FEAR IF YOU DON'T TAKE IT, YOU'LL DAMAGE YOUR MIND AND SPIRIT.

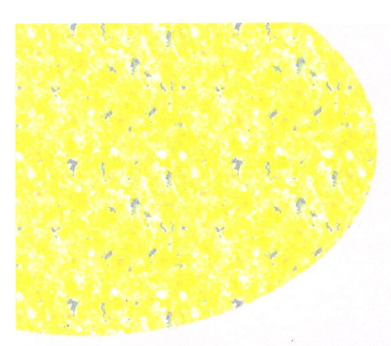

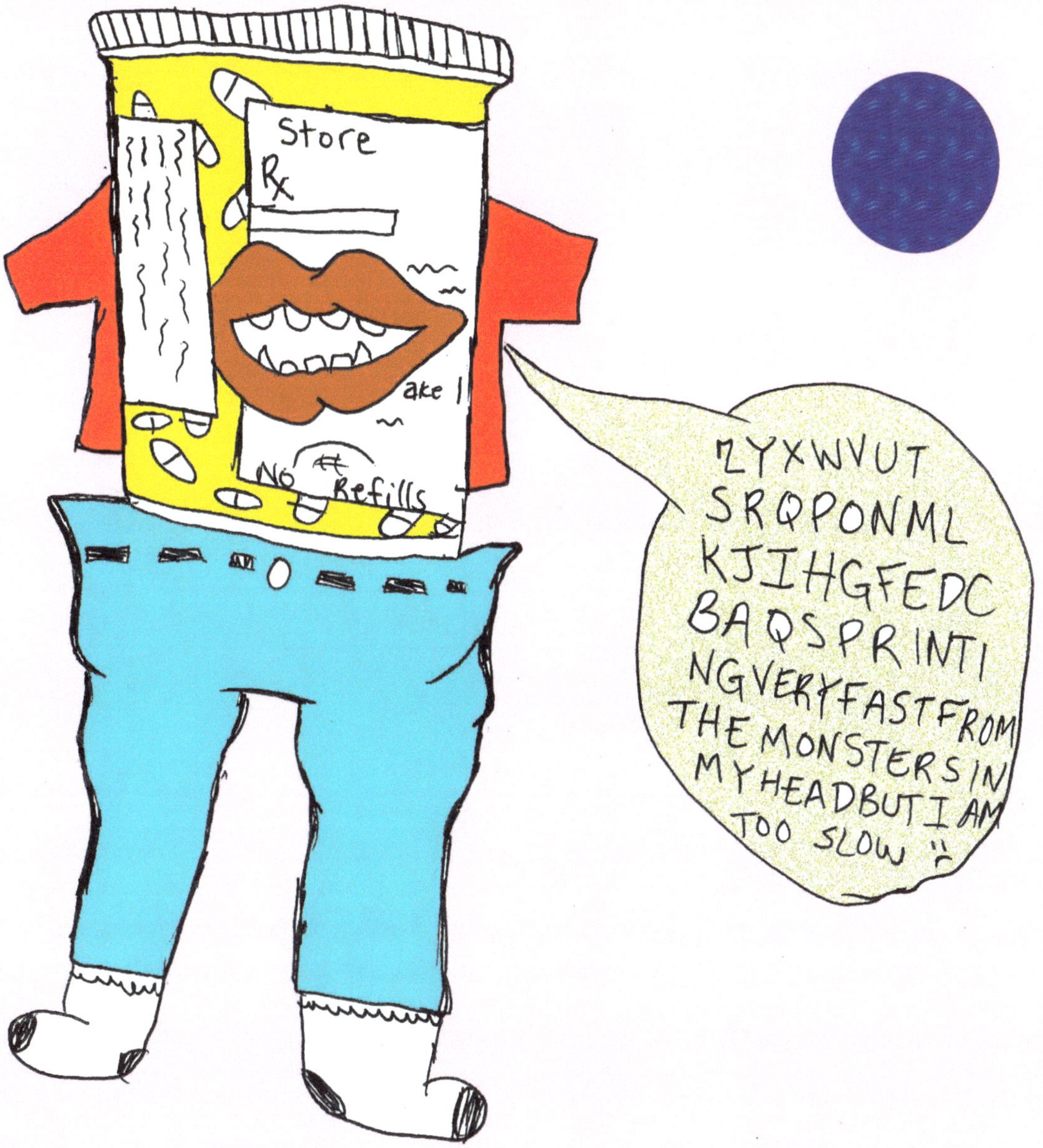

FUDGEWILLI

TAKE YOUR MEDICINE EDDY

JEFFERSON, PLEASE BE

CAUTIOUS OF YOUR CHOICES

IF YOU TOOK ALL OF YOUR

MEDS THEN YOU WOULDN'T

HEAR THOSE VOICES.

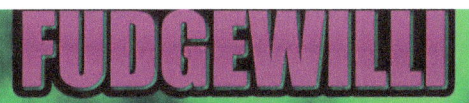
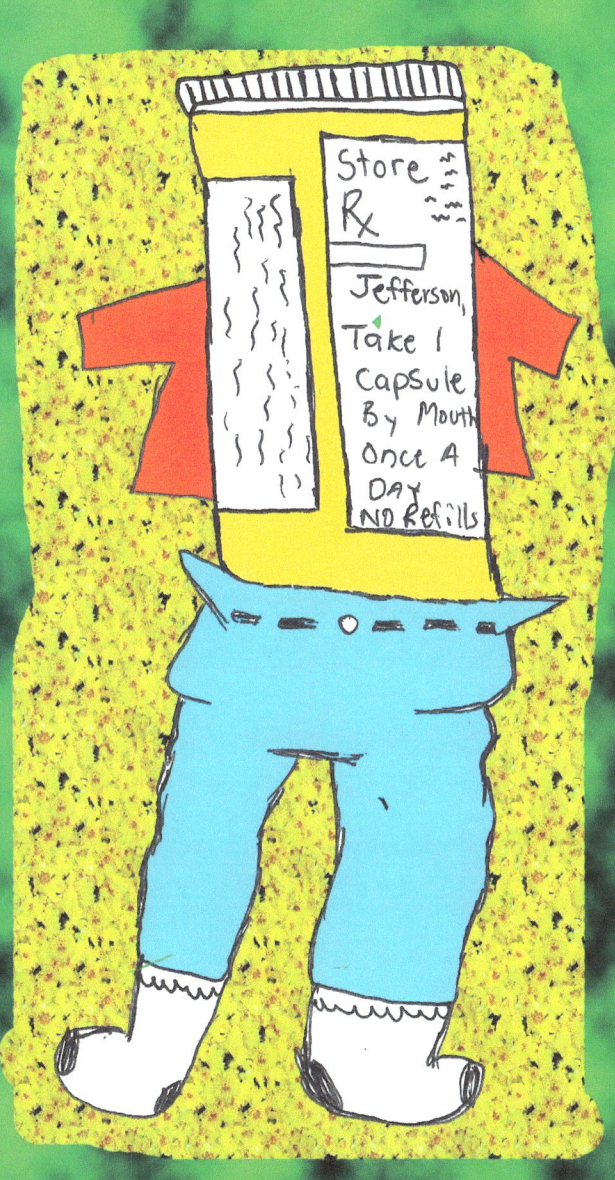

TAKE YOUR MEDICINE EDDY JEFFERSON, IT SHOULDNT BE SOMETHING TO AVOID. YOU SHOULD ACTUALLY WANT TO TAKE IT, SO YOU WONT BE PARANOID.

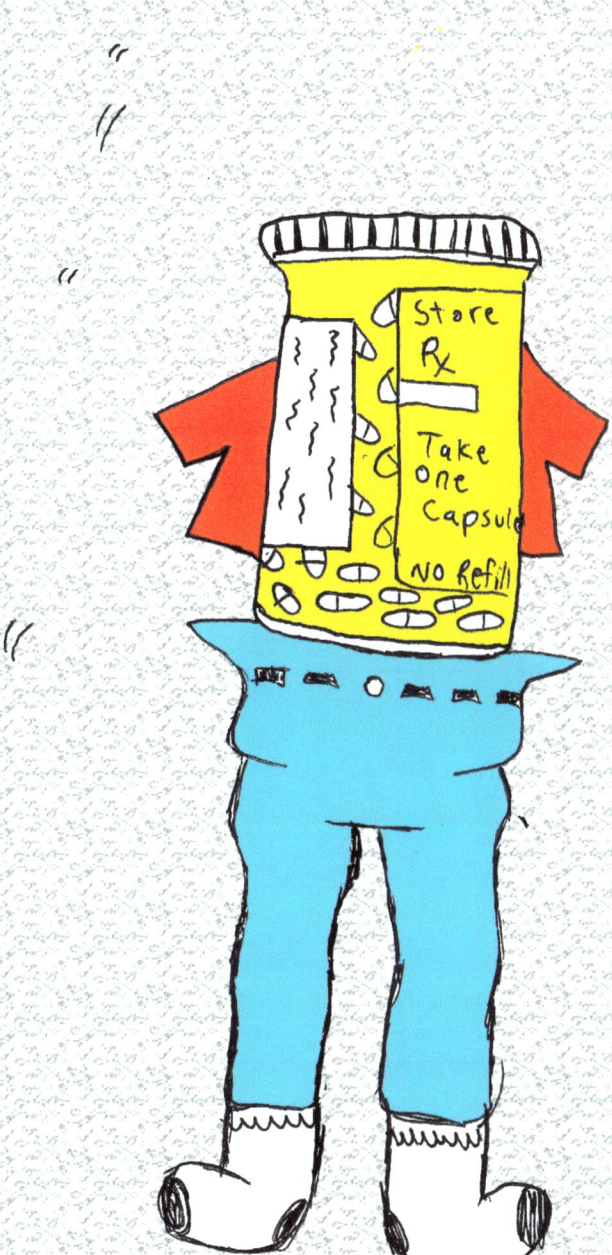

FUDGEWILLI

TAKE YOUR MEDICINE EDDY JEFFERSON, YOU'RE NOT ACTING LIKE YOURSELF. I'M CONCERNED FOR YOUR WELL BEING ALSO FOR YOUR MENTAL HEALTH.

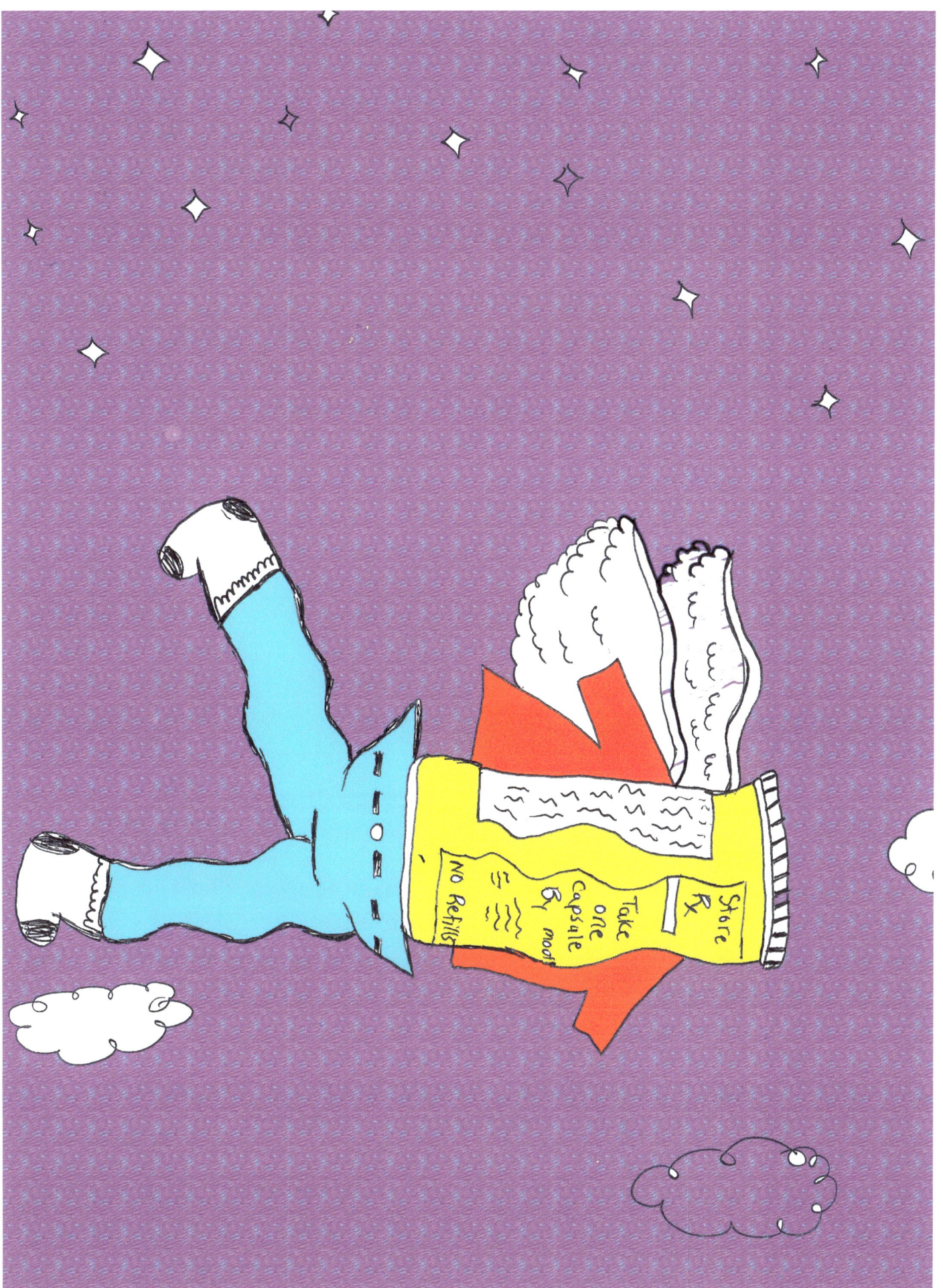

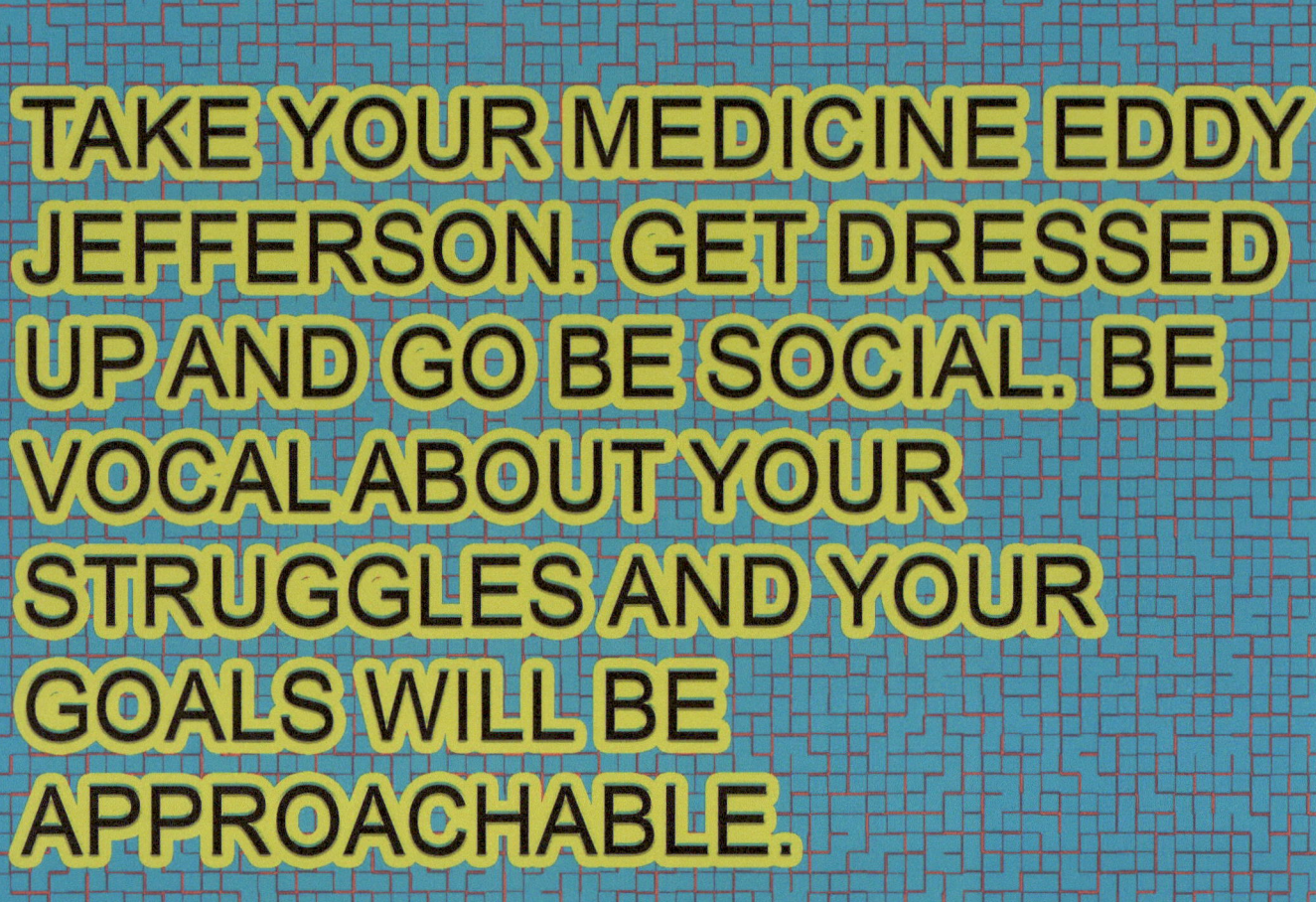

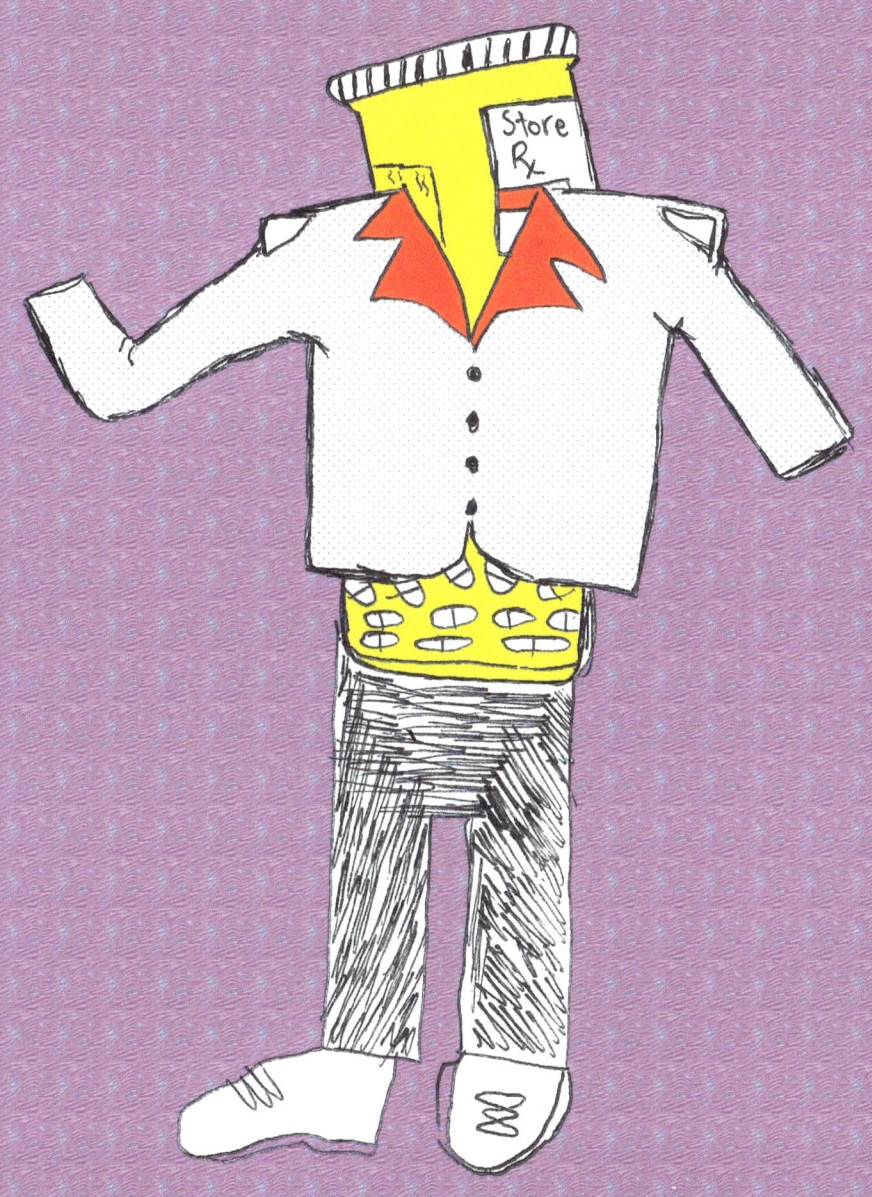

FUDGEWILLI

TAKE YOUR MEDICINE

EDDY JEFFERSON, WHEN

YOU DONT TAKE IT I CAN TELL.

I JUST WANT YOU TO BE

HEALTHY AND I WANT YOU TO

DO WELL.

FUDGEWILLI

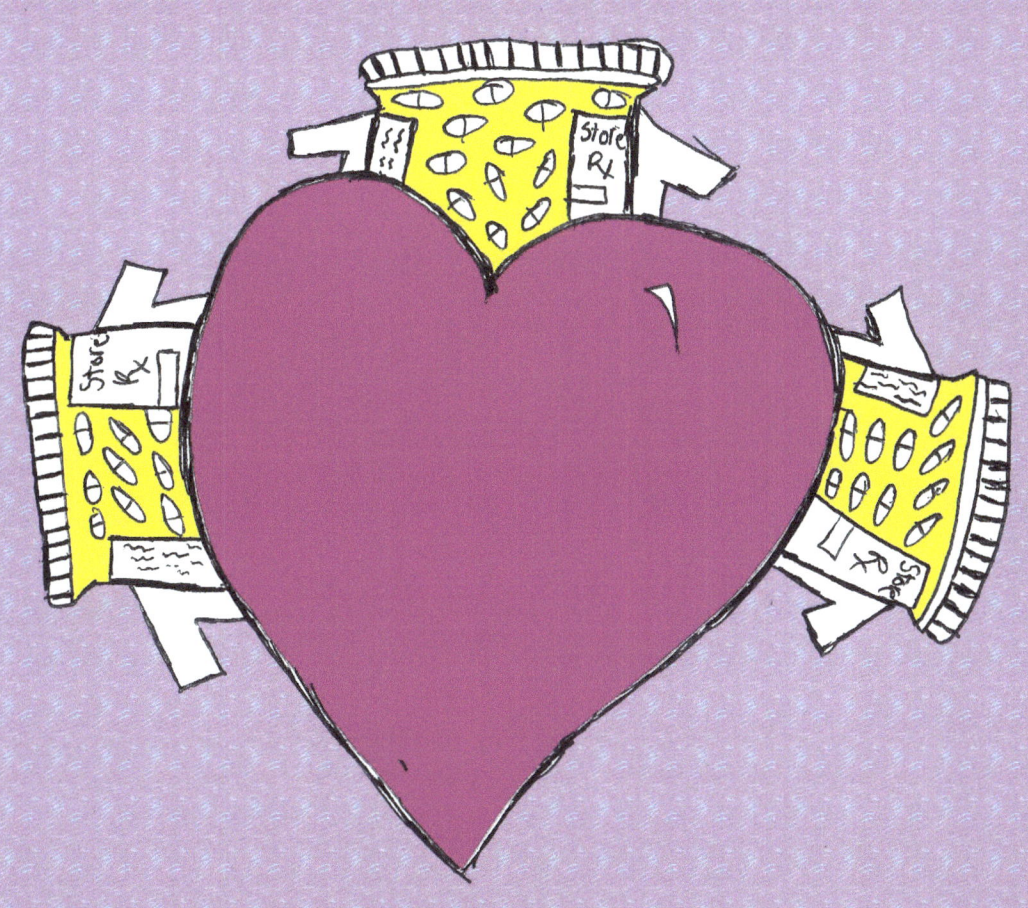

TAKE YOUR MEDICINE EDDY JEFFERSON. NO ONE'S FOLLOWING YOU AROUND. AND THERE'S NO NEED TO HOLD YOUR EARS BEACAUSE THERE ARE NOT ANY SOUNDS

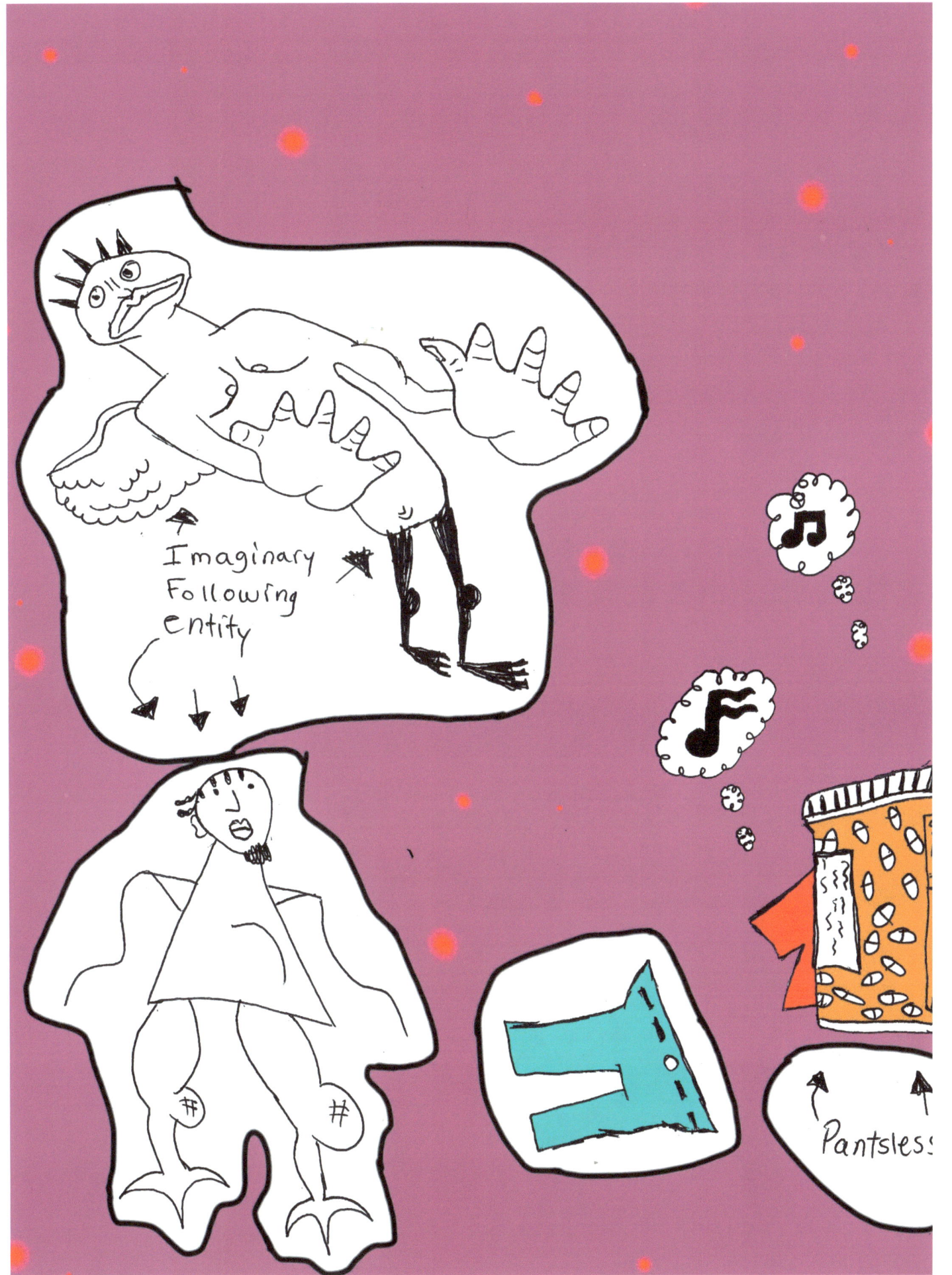

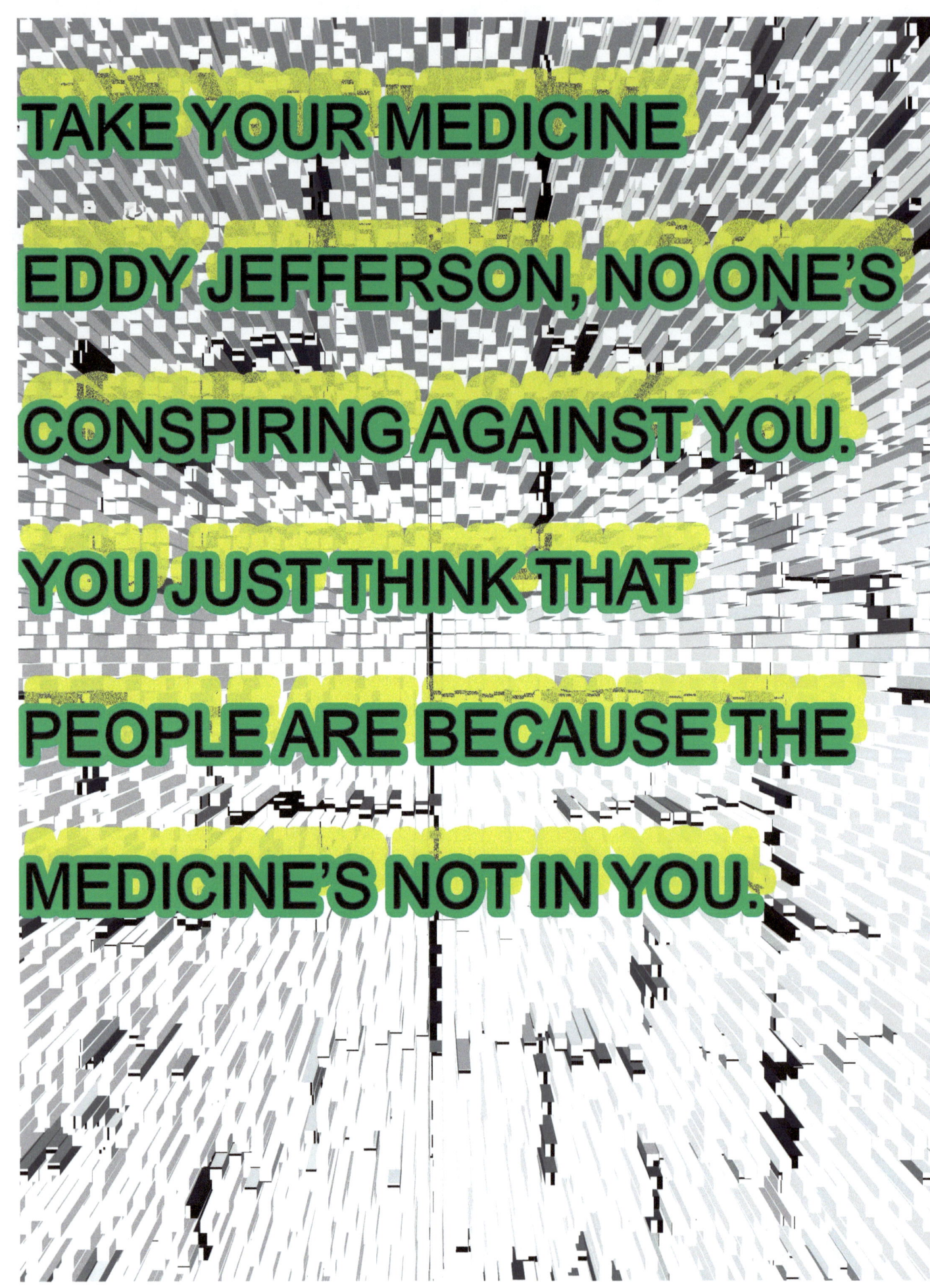

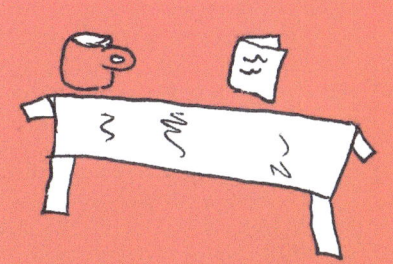
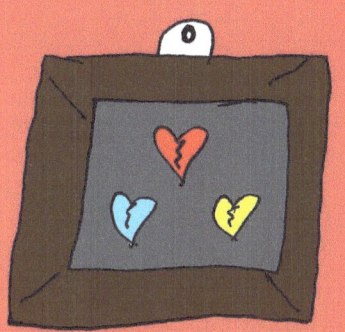
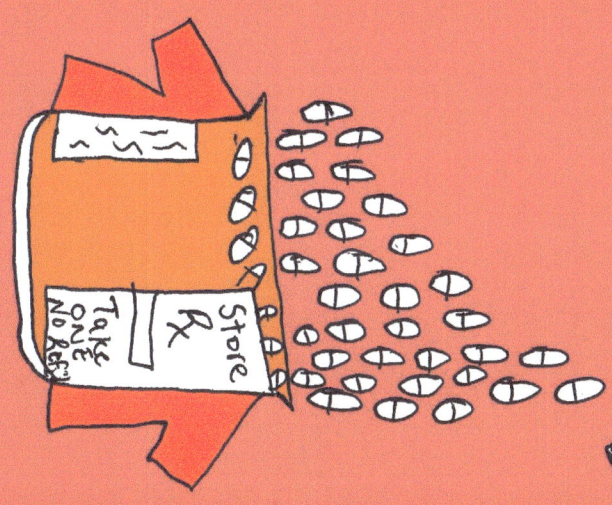
Spilled Pills
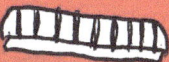

TAKE YOUR MEDICINE EDDY JEFFERSON. YOUR BEHAVIOR ITS JUST SCARING ME. SO BE SURE TO BE OPEN ON YOUR NEXT VISIT TO THERAPY.

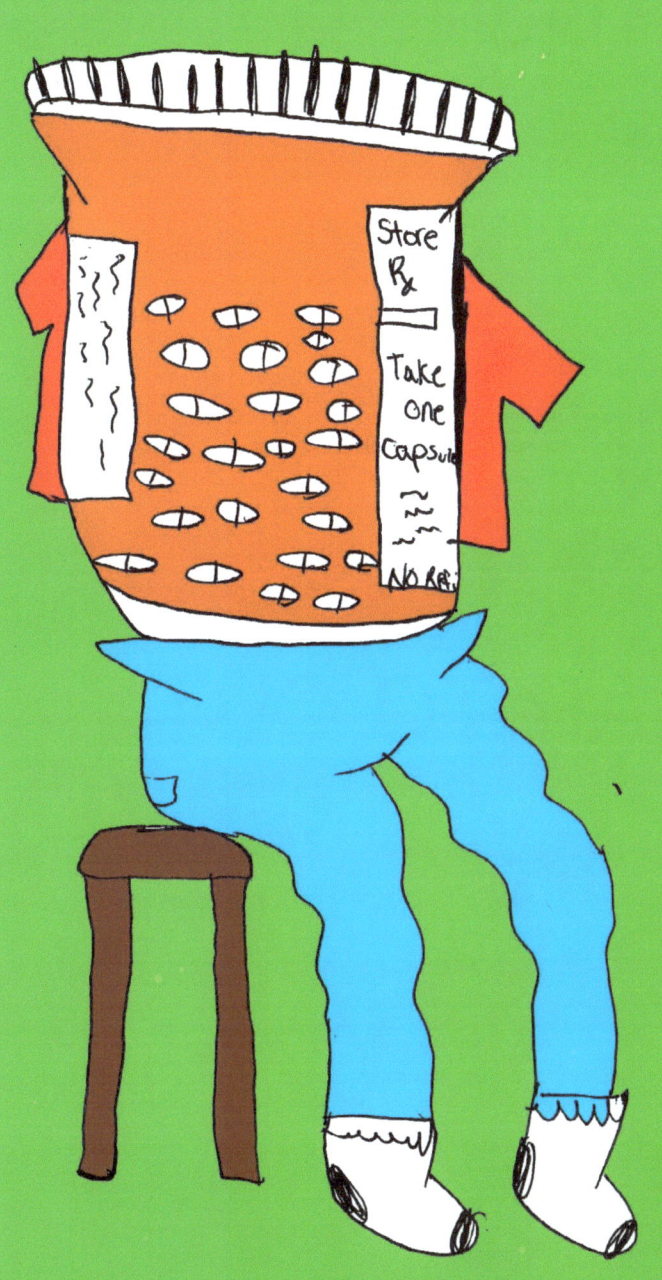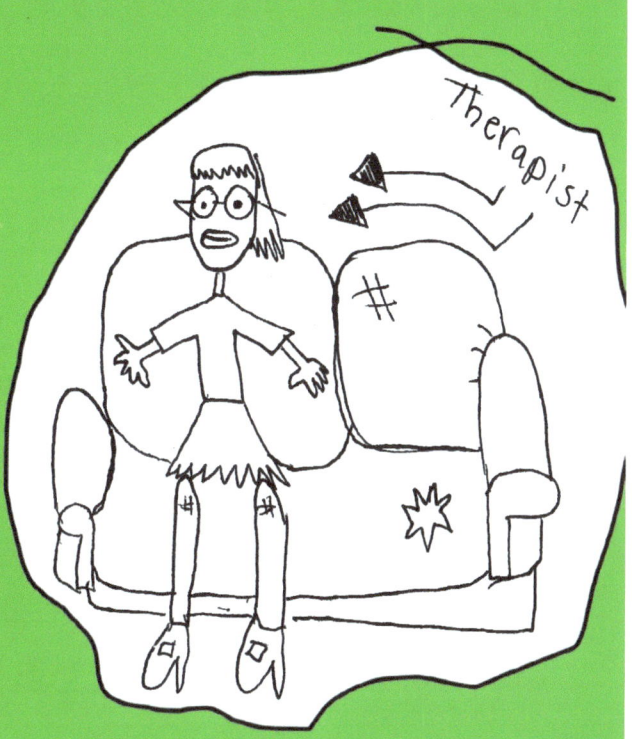

TAKE YOUR MEDICINE EDDY JEFFERSON, I KNOW IT ISN'T FAIR BUT I KNOW YOU HAVEN'T TAKEN IT BECAUSE YOU PAID AN EAR TO CUT YOUR HAIR

FUDGEWILLI

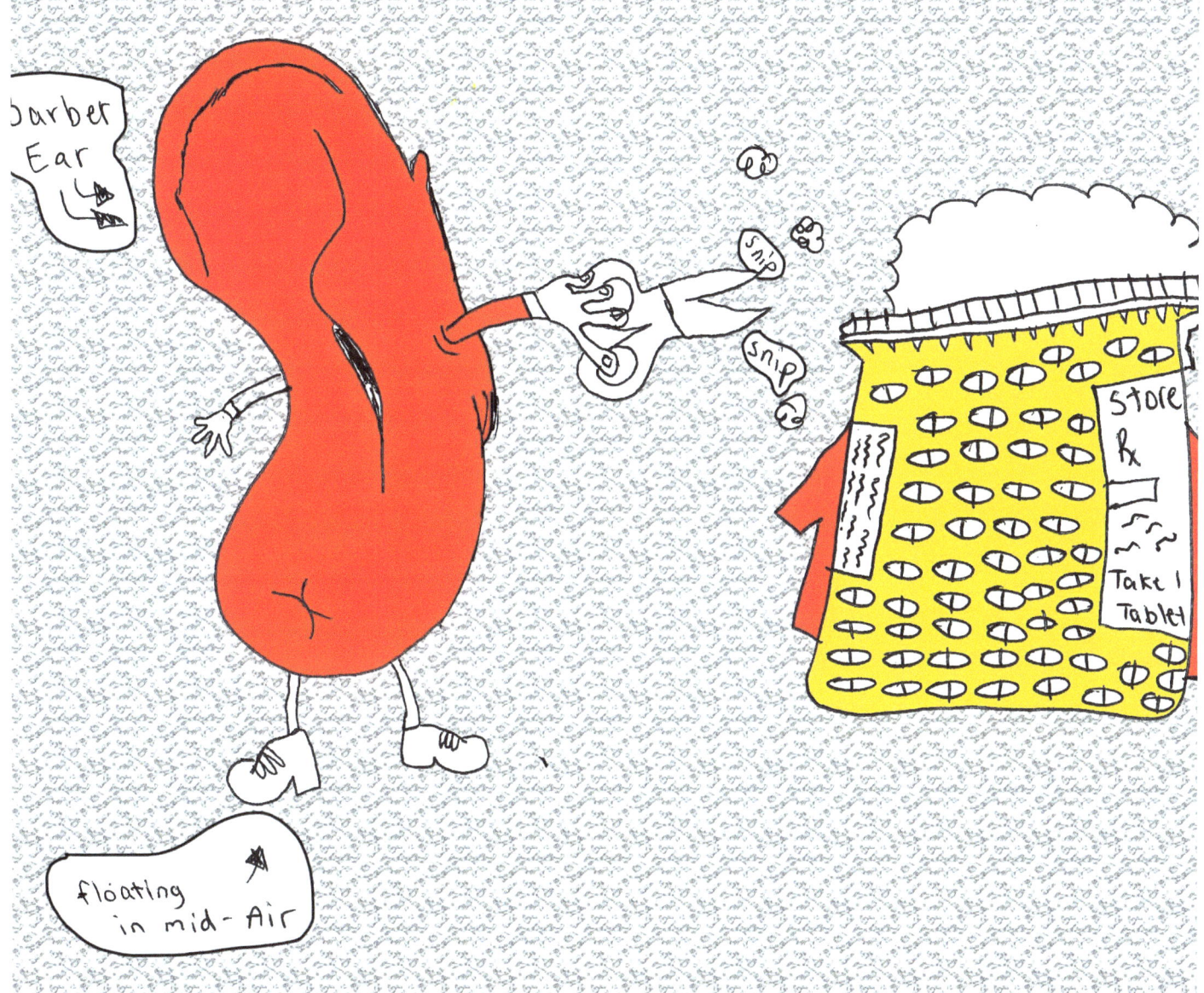

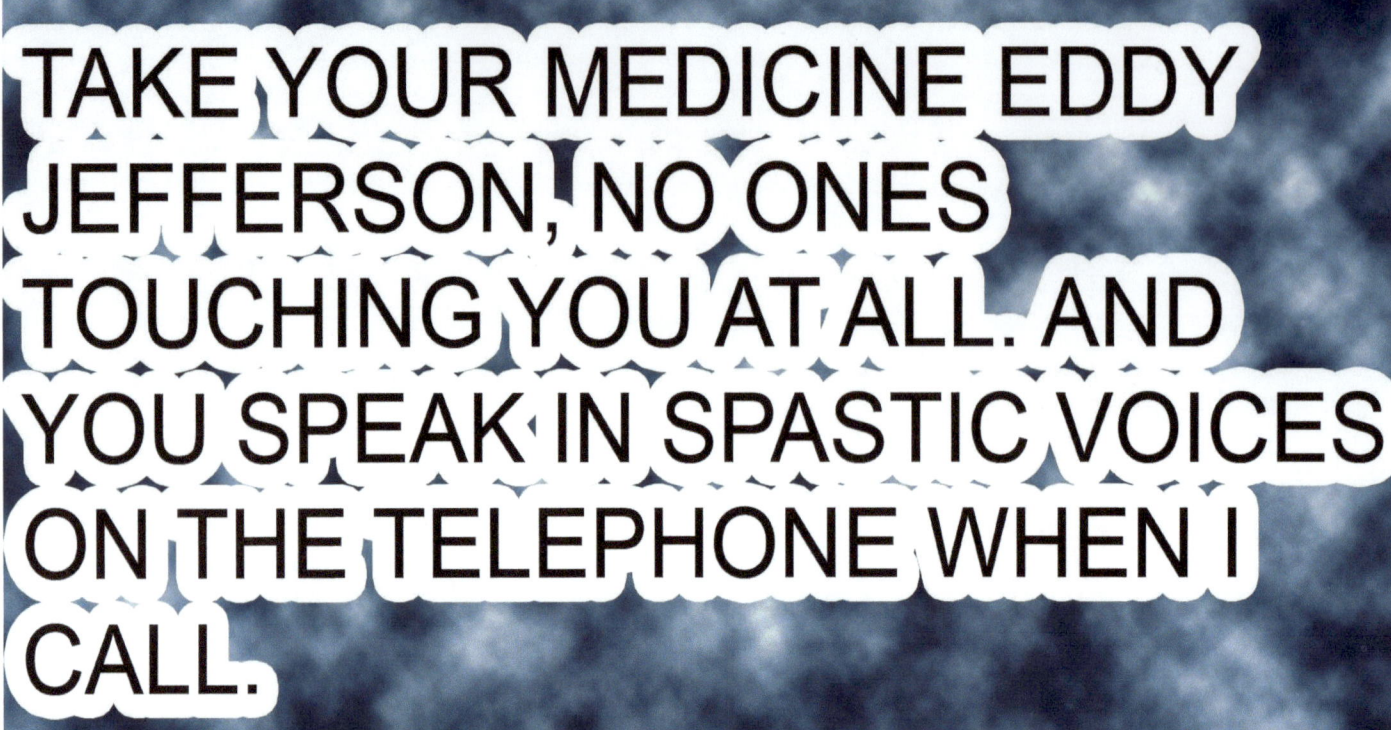

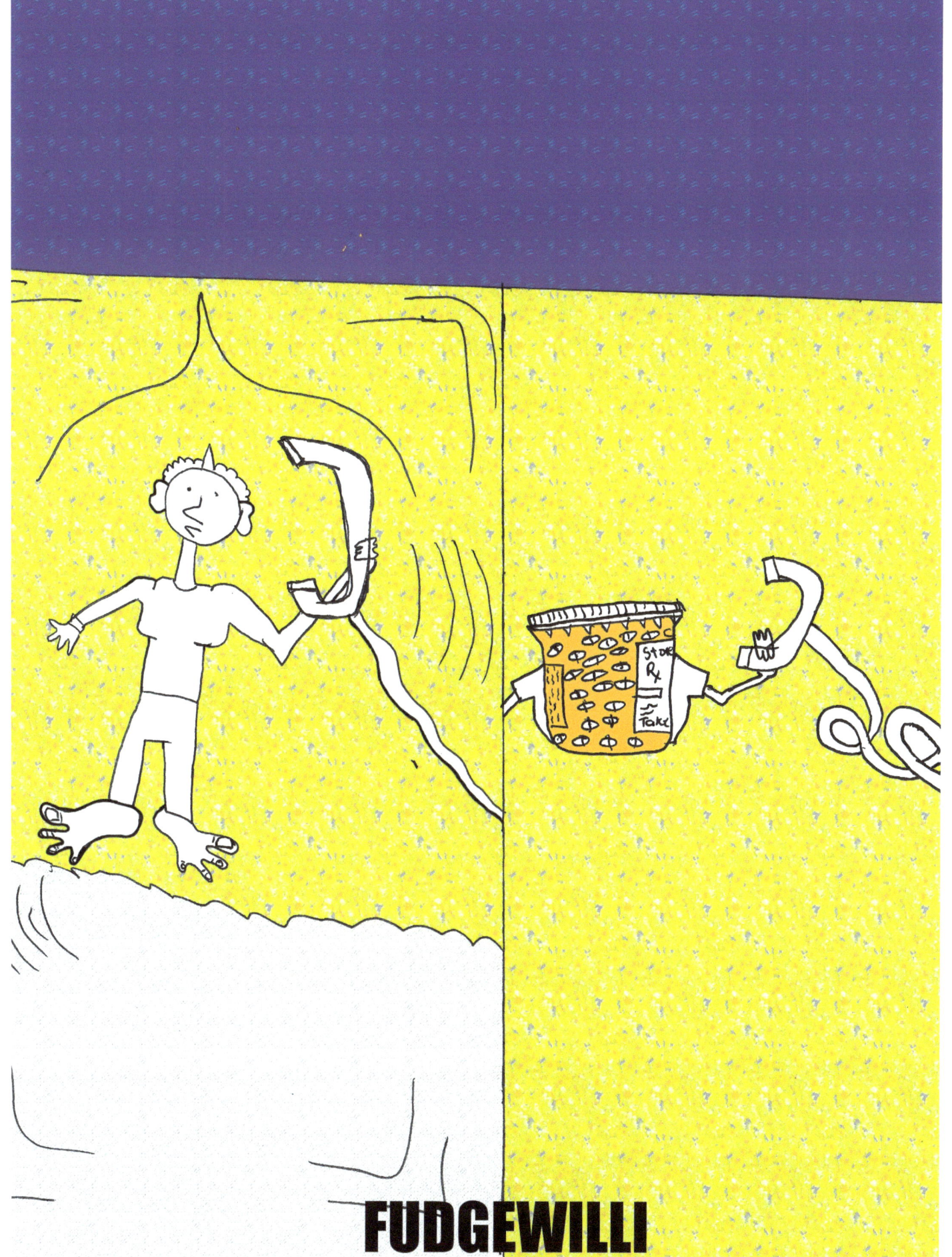

FUDGEWILLI

TAKE YOUR MEDICINE EDDY JEFFERSON, HOW'D YOUR MOOD SO QUICKLY CHANGE? I UNDERSTAND YOU EDDY JEFFERSON, YOU'RE NOT WEIRD OR DERANGED

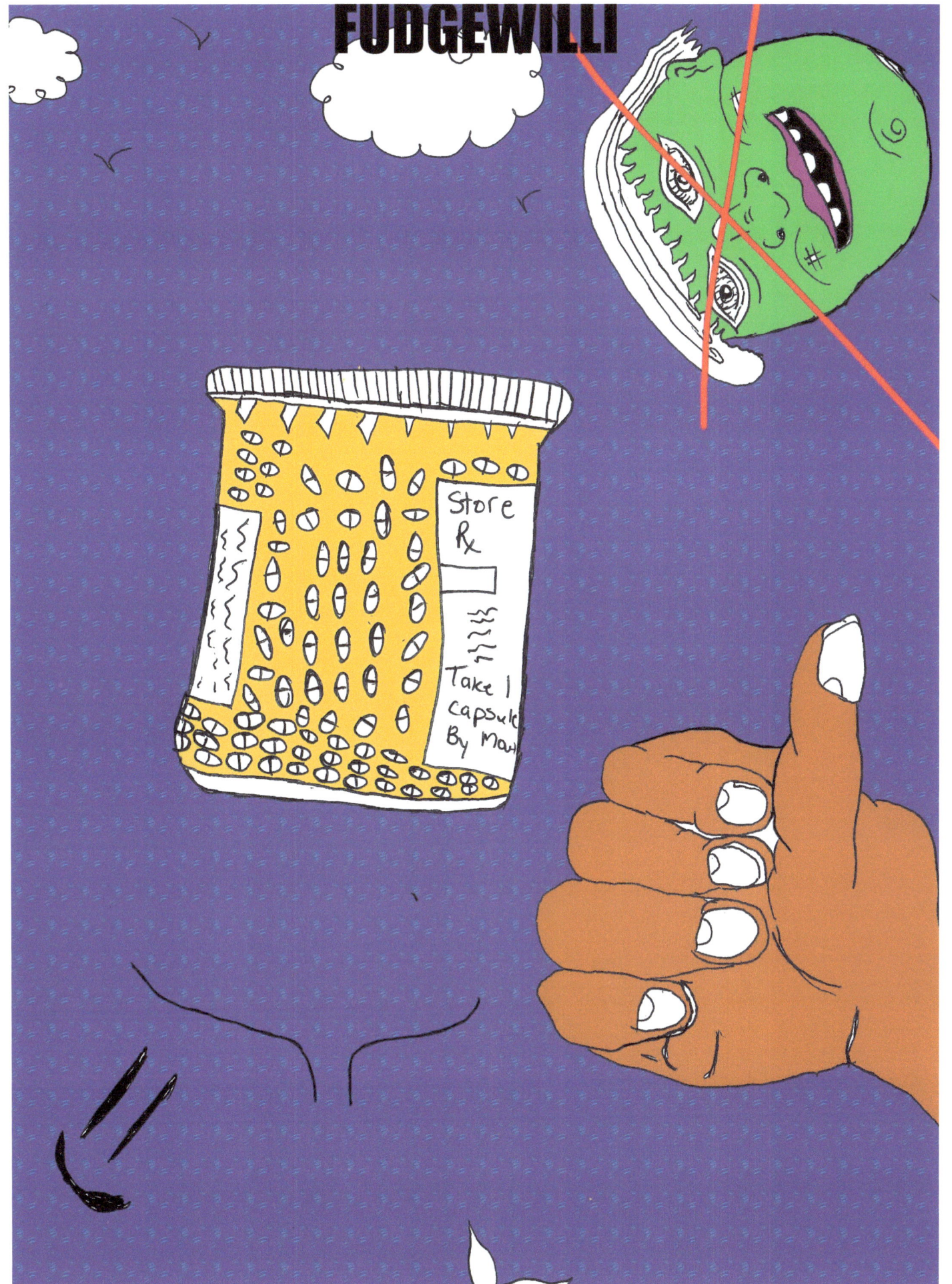

TAKE YOUR MEDICINE EDDY JEFFERSON, WE ALL LOVE YOU AND YOU KNOW THIS. WE'RE ALL ROOTING FOR YOU TO CONQUER THIS BATTLE WITH PSYCHOSIS.

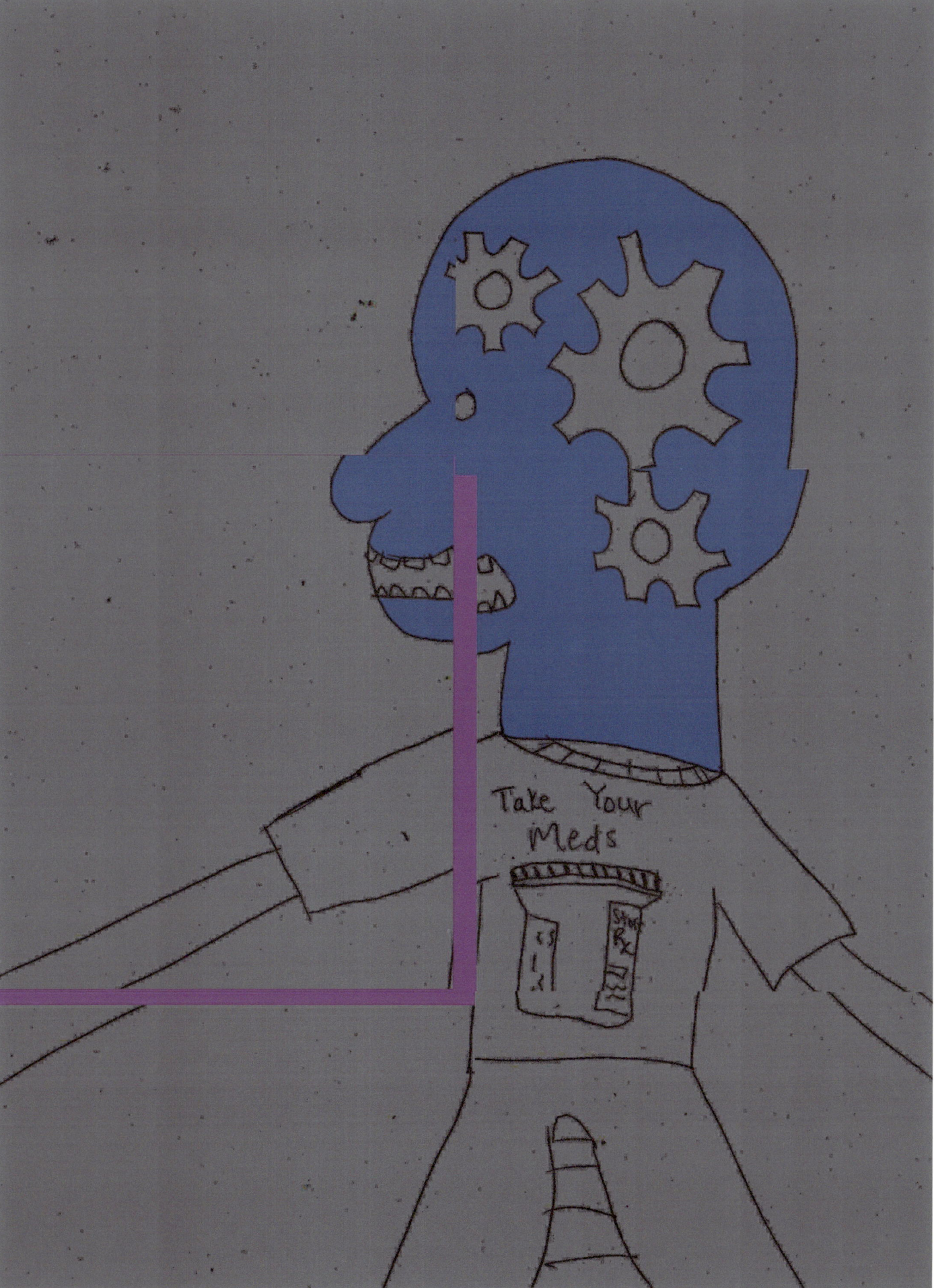